CHANGE THE WAY YOU THINK

180 YOUR THOUGHTS

Become The Woman You Always Knew You Could Be

GINA SIMS

Table of Contents

Chapter 1:

How To Simplify Your Life And Maximise Your Results

The word "simplicity" seems almost like a single-word oxymoron. The fast-paced, tech-driven world we live in makes it almost impossible to keep it simple. More and more apps are created every day to help make daily tasks such as communicating, shopping, and budgeting simpler – but the truth is, life these days couldn't be more complex.

We can agree that on most days, 24 hours just isn't enough time to get it all done, even though our multi-tasking skills are at their max. There is a widespread *need* for a simpler routine, but achieving success where that's concerned, is complicated. Where do you even start? (See, even the first step is hard!)

The Pareto principle, commonly known as the 80/20 rule, is a rule that has been universally accepted to explain the balance of output vs. input. The 80/20 rule states that 80% of results come from 20% of the action in a simple sentence. The 80/20 rule has proven to be true time and time again in many aspects of business such as economics, sales, real estate, health and safety, information technology, and sports.

How does this apply to you? It boils down to 80% of overall output -or- your accomplishments, at home, at work, in the gym, etc., comes from 20% of input -or- focused time, energy, and effort. So, in other words, to make the simplest and most effective strides to your goals, you have to focus on the *right* 20%. Clear as mud? Okay, let's look at an example. Have you ever known someone who tends to keep busy all the time but never really gets anything accomplished? That is because they are taking the path of least resistance, working on lots of little things that don't have a high value or return. Prioritizing quick, trivial, or less effective tasks over more difficult, time-consuming, yet impactful tasks is the procrastination paradox that leads to running in circles but never getting things done.

What's the solution? Goal prioritization and time management. Try this exercise to help simplify your goal and task list down to what matters to you.

1. Make a list of 10 things you want to accomplish in the next 30 days – in no particular order. These ten goals can apply to any area of your life – personal or professional. (The first of a new month is a great time to try this for the first time.)

2. Assign a category to each goal – family/friends, career, personal, etc.

3. Review the list carefully, considering the areas of your life each goal will impact. Now rank these 10 goals from 1-10; 1 = most important, 10 = least important.

If you are going to take Bruce Lee's path to simplicity by "hacking away at the unessential," – first determine what *is essential* (AKA rank your goals and priorities) and then start to remove the small barriers in your path that you can control.

Chapter 2:

Successful People Start Before They Feel Ready

We all have humble beginnings. We all start from the womb of our mothers, living the same baby life everyone else has lived before us, and everyone after us will.

We get our lives as our parents serve them to us. They send us to get the education and sometimes we have to make those arrangements for ourselves. Sometimes we get the food hot and good-looking just being served to us without even wanting to ask for it.

But life isn't always this kind and caring.

How many times do we wish for things like I will do this better tomorrow, I will get that someday, I have to look for a better job, I have to do something about the extra weight that I am carrying.

We all have a wish list and it is always growing. But rarely do we do something about them. We always go back to our normal life and don't do anything about it as we always have. Sounds familiar?

It is the reality and the curse of living in this time of having everything we can wish so never wanting to struggle for other things.

There might be a lot of reasons for every one of us for not trying, or trying but not getting what we want.

We lag in a lot of things and there are hundreds of explanations for them, but the most common is the 'FEAR'.

Fear of rejection, fear of waiting, fear of not being good enough, fear of the unknown, and mostly fear of starting something from scratch. All these fears are legitimate and justifiable, but you are not getting much by fear either. So why not be fearless and actually start doing something?

We have a lot on our plate and we all have our bad days, but to start fresh, you don't need fear or an indicator or vision, you just need the tiniest of motivation that you have to make something for yourself and you and only you are your sole driving force.

Things will start happening for you one time or the other. You only need to maintain vigor at any age you are.

You don't have a set path. Don't think that you will get mature and stable once you hit the 30's or middle age. Time will not set the path for you. You, yourself have to set the time straight.

You don't need to be 30 to be mature, you can be 15 and still be a much mature and emotionally stable person than the one who has 5 children.

Your life is in your hands and you have a responsibility towards yourself from the time you get a hold of your senses. Because you are always ready to turn things around.

You don't need to feel ready, but you need to show yourself that you were ready all along by just jumping into the pond of opportunities and the world will open its treasury for you.

You don't need to be perfect to start, but you need to start to be perfect!

Chapter 3:

Don't Live Your Life In Regret

Take this for a lesson today; There is no greater pain than that of regret.

Hopelessness is one thing that can crack a soul, but nothing is more hurting than that of lifelong regret. We take up things in our life that we deem helpful for the times to come. But never do we ever take risks, just because we want to have a smooth uncomplicated life.

Life was never meant to be lived as reading off a paper. Neither can you expect it to be a smooth walk on a beach? There are always some pebbles on the way and always some hedges where you need to twist and turn to fit and climb.

We all will eventually o through a period of endless questioning where we judge our every step and every decision whether if it was bad or not good enough!

But why are we indulging in this waste of time when we have so much better things to do right now in this present time slot.

When you are on a long journey, nothing will make sense. When you are on your path to greatness, you will always look back and get drawn back a little every time.

But once you reach the top, you will have a final look back into your past and everything will make sense in a split second.

Life is a roller coaster and we all have baggage. We must have because no one can have lived a long life and have a straight, plain, and colorless script where nothing happened out of the ordinary.

The uncertainty of life is what defines life to its true reality.

We, humans, are a combination of deterministic and non-deterministic behavior where we get triggered on thoughts of shame and failure but rarely do we learn to listen to those failures and try to change our habits.

Things have a course of happening and we always get behind the things that take most of us down the lane. That is where we feel the walk of shame and remember the feeling for the rest of our life.

But why do we feel the urge to remain connected to our shameful past? What needs do we have with feeling shame? Why do we need to remember and regret the things that the world has forgotten a long time ago? Why do we need to keep those memories alive?

A billion incidents are happening every second and we try to keep all our baggage with us till the day we take it with us to our graves.

What we should be doing is to forgive everyone and especially ourselves, to release some positive energy and make some space for the happy times that are to come.

We should let those happy moments erase all our regrets and ease our path for the best future that time could ever earn us. But what you should do ultimately, is to regret what you haven't done yet, rather than what you have done!

Chapter 4:

Five Ways To Control Your Thoughts

The power of thoughts.

Thoughts are very powerful because they greatly influence the direction our lives take. Our failures and successes are anchored on our thinking patterns. We score big in life when we learn how to dominate our minds and submit them to our desires.

The greater the external influence on our decisions, the more likely we lose control of our thoughts. Here are five ways to control your thoughts:

1. Meditation.

It is the ability to reflect deeply on the occurrences in your life. Meditation is taking a deep reflective introspect of your life. Sometimes we need to take a break from our busy schedules and look back at the far we have come from. The journey we have walked hitherto shall inspire us to confidently move into the future.

Meditation is often perceived as old-fashioned because it is very basic. It appears unattractive but once you learn to do it in the right way, there is no turning back. Do not mistake it for idleness or wishful thinking because it is neither of them.

It begins with a mental walk down memory lane. You count your blessings one after another and take stock of your achievements. You can consolidate your thoughts through meditation as you plan for your next move. Meditation provides room for mental growth because you are free from any pressure to act therein.

2. Taking feedback.

How is feedback related to controlling our thoughts? There is a strong connection between the two. We live in a social world where interaction with different types of people is inevitable. Their perceptions and the doctrines they believe also vary. The people we live amongst are the mirror in which we can look at ourselves.

Strangers, friends, and family are very important circles that we surround ourselves with. Apart from strangers, our family and friends have been with us long enough to understand our thinking patterns. Their feedback about our decisions on various issues is very important because we can control our thoughts bordering on their suggestions.

We should learn to take feedback even from strangers we interact with briefly. They could make very important observations on our intellectuality which could spell the turning point of our thoughts. The power of feedback should not be underrated.

3. Taking a SWOT analysis.

We may have considered a SWOT analysis on our businesses but not on ourselves. If it is good for business, why is it not for ourselves? Our thoughts need to be audited from time to time for us to identify the red flags within. We can thereafter act from a point of knowledge because we understand our strengths and weaknesses even better.

We can work to improve our weaknesses and fortify our strengths in thoughts when we analyze them thoroughly. We can program our thoughts when we understand our personalities better.

A SWOT analysis enables us to identify the red zones we should not enter because they could spell doom for us. We also learn the limits we should not exceed because they threaten to disrupt our good thoughts. We operate within a healthy framework that our minds flourish.

4. Submitting to spiritual authority.

It is good to subscribe to a belief or religion. Every religion has its practices that are beyond physical comprehension if your heart and thoughts are left out. The beauty of religious beliefs is its mystery in understanding the spirituality concepts around them.

Religion reinforces morality and upright thinking. Religious people train their thoughts within the confines of their beliefs. This enables them to be disciplined and control their thoughts not to stray away from the values they practice.

Religion rebukes evil thoughts and promotes the good ones. It is the prefect of upright thinking and curbs many evils before they even happen. If you have a problem with having your thoughts under control, consider joining a religion.

5. Consider the fear of the unknown.

Fear is destructive when misused but very constructive when channeled correctly. The fear of the unknown is a limiting factor to very many things. Over the years, humanity has restrained itself from acting or thinking against acceptable societal norms because of the fear of the unknown that lies beyond.

You can bring your thoughts to submission when you consider the red zones that you should not approach, even in your mind. Your thinking will be disciplined not to stray into unchartered territories because of untold consequences.

In conclusion, controlling our thoughts is a big win if we at all want to be successful. These five ways are effective in bringing your thoughts to submission.

Chapter 5:

4 Ways Geniuses Come Up with Great Ideas

Following are thumbnail descriptions of strategies common to the thinking styles of creative geniuses in science, art, and industry throughout history.

1. **Geniuses Look at Problems in Many Different Ways**

Genius often comes from finding a new perspective that no one else has taken. Leonardo da Vinci believed that to gain knowledge about the form of problems, you begin by learning how to restructure them in many different ways. He felt the first way he looked at a problem was too biased toward his usual way of seeing things. He would restructure his problem by looking at it from one perspective and move to another view and still another. With each move, his understanding would deepen, and he would begin to understand the essence of the problem. Einstein's theory of relativity is, in essence, a description of the interaction between different perspectives. Freud's analytical methods were designed to find details that did not fit with traditional perspectives to find a completely new point of view.

In order to creatively solve a problem, the thinker must abandon the initial approach that stems from past experience and re-conceptualize the problem. By not settling with one perspective, geniuses do not merely solve existing problems, like inventing an environmentally friendly fuel. They identify new ones. It does not take a genius to analyze dreams; it required Freud to ask in the first place what meaning dreams carry from our psyche.

2. Geniuses Make Their Thoughts Visible

The explosion of creativity in the Renaissance was intimately tied to the recording and conveying of a vast knowledge in a parallel language, a language of drawings, graphs, and diagrams — as, for instance, in the renowned diagrams of DaVinci and Galileo. Galileo revolutionized science by making his thought visible with charts, maps, and drawings, while his contemporaries used conventional mathematical and verbal approaches.

Once geniuses obtain a certain minimal verbal facility, they seem to develop a skill in visual and spatial abilities, which gives them the flexibility to display information in different ways. When Einstein had thought through a problem, he always found it necessary to formulate his subject in as many different ways as possible, including diagrammatically. He had a very visual mind. He thought in terms of visual and spatial forms rather than thinking along purely mathematical or verbal lines of reasoning. In fact, he believed that words and numbers, as they are written or spoken, did not play a significant role in his thinking process.

3. Geniuses Produce

A distinguishing characteristic of genius is immense productivity. Thomas Edison held 1,093 patents, still the record. He guaranteed productivity by giving himself and his assistants' idea quotas. His own personal quota was one minor invention every ten days and a major innovation every six months. Bach wrote a cantata every week, even when he was sick or exhausted. Mozart produced more than six hundred pieces of music. Einstein is best known for his paper on relativity, but he published 248 other papers. T. S. Elliot's numerous drafts of "The Waste Land" constitute a jumble of good and bad passages that eventually was turned into a masterpiece. In a study of 2,036 scientists throughout history, Dean Kean Simonton of the University of California, Davis found that the most respected produced great works and more "bad" ones. Out of their massive quantity of work came quality. Geniuses produce. Period.

4. Geniuses Make Novel Combinations

Dean Keith Simonton, in his 1989 book Scientific Genius suggests that geniuses are geniuses because they form more novel combinations than the merely talented. His theory has etymology behind it: cogito — "I think — originally connoted "shake together": intelligent the root of "intelligence" means to "select among." This is a clear early intuition about the utility of permitting ideas and thoughts to randomly combine with each other and the utility of selecting from the many the few to retain. Like the highly playful child with a pailful of Legos, a genius constantly combines and recombines ideas, images, and thoughts into different combinations in their conscious and subconscious minds. Consider Einstein's equation, $E=mc2$. Einstein did not invent the concepts of energy, mass, or speed of light. Instead, by combining these concepts in a novel way, he could look at the same world as everyone else and see something different. The laws of heredity on which the modern science of genetics is based are the results of Gregor Mendel, who combined mathematics and biology to create new science.

Chapter 6:

Five Habits of A Healthy Lifestyle

A healthy lifestyle is everybody's dream. The young and old, rich and poor, weak and strong, and male and female all want a happily ever after and many years full of life. The price to pay to achieve this dream is what distinguishes all these classes of people. What are you ready to forego as the opportunity cost to have a healthy lifestyle?

Here are five habits for a healthy lifestyle.

1.   Eating Healthy Food

Your health is heavily dependent on your diet. You have heard that what goes inside a man does not defile him, but what goes out of him does. In this case, the opposite is true. What a man takes as food or beverage affects him directly. It can alter the body's metabolism and introduce toxins in the body hence endangering his life.

Most people do not take care of what they feed on. They eat anything edible that is readily available without any consideration. All other factors like the nutritive value of the food and its hygiene are secondary to most modern people who have thrown caution to the wind. Towns and cities are full of fast food joints and attract masses from all over. It is the most lucrative business these days. Are these fast foods healthy?

As much as the hygiene could be up to standards (due to the measures put in place by authorities), the composition of these foods (mostly chips and broiler chicken) is wanting. The cooking oil used is full of cholesterol that is a major cause of cardiac diseases. To lead a healthy lifestyle, eating healthy food should be a priority.

2. Regular Exercising

The human body requires regular exercise to be fit. Running, walking, swimming, or going to the gym are a few of the many ways that people can exercise. It is a call to get out of your comfort zone to ward off some lifestyle diseases. It is often misconstrued that exercising is a reserve for sportsmen and women. This fallacy has taken root in the minds of many people.

Unlearn the myths about exercises that have made most people shun them. The benefits of exercising are uncountable. It improves pressure and blood circulation in the body. Exercises also burn excess calories in tissues that would otherwise clog blood vessels and pose a health hazard. Research has shown that most people who exercise are healthy and fall sick less often. This is everyone's dream but the few who choose to pay the price enjoy it. Choose to be healthy by doing away with frequent motor vehicle transport and instead walk. A simple walk is an exercise already. When you fail to exercise early enough, you will be a frequent patient at the hospital. Prevention is always better than cure.

In the words of world marathon champion, Eliud Kipchoge, a running nation is a healthy nation.

3. Regular Medical Checkup

When was the last time you went for a medical checkup even when you were not sick? If the answer is negative or a long time ago, then a healthy lifestyle is still unreachable. A medical examination will reveal any disease in its early stages.

In most third-world countries, healthcare systems are not fully developed. Its citizens only go to the hospital when a disease has progressed and is in its late stages. At such a time, there is a higher probability of the patient succumbing to it. Doctors advise people to seek medical attention at the slightest symptom to treat and manage long-term illnesses. Regular medical checkups help one become more productive at work.

Is a healthy lifestyle attainable? Yes, it is when one takes the necessary measures to fight diseases. Regular medical checkups can be financially draining. Seek an insurance policy that can underwrite your health risks and this will make medical expenses affordable.

4. Staying Positive

A bad attitude is like a flat tire. If you do not change it, you will never go anywhere. There is a hidden power in having a positive attitude towards life. It all starts in the mind. When you conceive the right attitude towards life, you have won half the battle.

A healthy lifestyle starts with the mind. If you believe it, you can achieve it. So limitless is the human mind that it strongly influences the direction of a person's life. As much as there are challenges in life, do not allow them to conquer your mind or take over your spirit. Once they do, you will be constantly waging a losing battle. Is that what we want?

Associate with positive like-minded people and you will be miles away from depression and low self-esteem. We all desire that healthy lifestyle.

5. Have A Confidant And A Best Friend

Who is a best friend? He/she is someone you can trust to share your joy and sadness, and your high and low moments. You should be careful in your selection of a confidant because it may have strong ramifications if the friendship is not genuine.

A confidant is someone you can confide in comfortably without fear of him/her leaking your secrets. He/she will help you overcome some difficult situations in life. We all need a shoulder to lean on in our darkest times and a voice to comfort us that it is darkest before dawn. This helps fortify our mental health. We grow better and stronger in this healthy lifestyle.

These are the five habits for a healthy lifestyle. When we live by them, success becomes our portion.

Chapter 7:

10 Habits of Jennifer Lawrence

Jennifer Lawrence is one of Hollywood's most famous actress, thanks to her role in films such as "The Hunger Games" and "Silver Linings Playbook." But, before her tremendous success, Lawrence struggled to build a name for herself as an actress and model in New York, where she moved when she was 14 years old. After breaking out as the tough-as-nails teenager Ree in the 2010 indie drama "Winter's Bone," Lawrence went on to star in multiple "X-Men" films and drama such as "American Hustle."

I can't think of anyone who doesn't adore Jennifer Lawrence. What is it about this actress that makes her so appealing? It's easy to list a thousand reasons to admire Jennifer Lawrence -from her incredible skill to her quick-witted humour- but honestly, the life lessons she attracts everyone to her.

Here are 10 life habits that Lawrence offers as lessons simply by being herself.

1. Strive for Health and Strength

"I'm never going to starve myself for a part," she declared on the cover of Elle in December 2012. "I don't want little girls to think, 'Oh, I want to look like Katniss; hence I'll skip meals." When you're trying to get your physique to appear just suitable, Emma on the other end is trying to make her body appear muscular and robust rather than skinny.

2. Refresh Yourself

How many times has Lawrence stumbled? That's what probably comes to your mind every time you see her trip over the hem of her gown at an awards presentation. Can anyone blame the girl for this? Those outfits appear to be impossible to walk in! But she trips, and every time, without fail, she gets back up and continues walking.

3. Accept Responsibility for Your Mistakes

Lawrence's awkward moments are all the more endearing because she is always the first to laugh at how clumsy she is when she stands. Remember when she collapsed at the 2013 Academy Awards? Or when she collapsed on the red carpet of the 2014 Academy Awards? What does it matter? We're all human, and J. Law never tries to hide it by acting cool and so should you.

4. The Truth Will Set You Free

Even if your truth seems to hurt more, such as that you pee very quickly or that your breasts are unequal, J. Law says that it is what it is, and to be anything other than herself isn't allowed. Embrace your flaws!

5. Look Past the Hype

Remember to key in what's genuine and what's not, and to keep your things in perspective, look past those who take themselves too seriously.

6. Maintain An Open Mind

Lawrence told E! News that her acting job will not bind her for the rest of her life. However, she understands that things happen and that people's lives change, and she is prepared to keep an open mind about it. Being open-minded will direct you to break the monotony for future possibilities.

7. Nobody Is Flawless

Can you recall a scene in American Hustle in which Lawrence's character discusses nail polish? Do you remember the nail polish? She claims it's the smell that keeps drawing her back since it's delicious on the outside but rotten on the inside. Not only is it a beautiful moment, but the discussion is a metaphor for everyone's good and evil sides. Nobody is flawless, and no one loves it when others claim to be.

8. Humility

During a BBC Radio 1 interview, Lawrence remarked her involvement in "The Hunger Games," where she genuinely adores watching the movies she makes because she gets to see how much of a troll, bad, and untalented is. Weird! Indeed, you wouldn't agree with her right? Bu she's adorable because she is humble.

9. Maintain a Sense of Humour

During an interview with Vogue, Lawrence sense of humour could be seen when she cracked a joke on how seeing 13-year olds give her nightmares. She effortlessly doesn't take life too seriously.

10. Love Your Body

Lawrence has spoken out numerous times about her body, challenging unrealistic beauty standards. She claimed in an interview with FLARE magazine that she would rather appear overweight on camera (and appear normal) than diet only to dress like a scarecrow. That is a whole lot of body positivity just for you!

Conclusion

Jennifer will teach you profound truths- when she acts, and when she put on a mask that conceals who she truly is. She given up none of her power by leaving the covers on the screen and refusing to act to "fit in" with Hollywood culture.

Chapter 8:

How to Value Being Alone

Some people are naturally happy alone. But for others, being solo is a challenge. If you fall into the latter group, there are ways to become more comfortable with being alone (yes, even if you're a hardcore extrovert).

Regardless of how you feel about being alone, building a good relationship with yourself is a worthy investment. After all, you *do* spend quite a bit of time with yourself, so you might as well learn to enjoy it.

Being alone isn't the same as being lonely.

Before getting into the different ways to find happiness in being alone, it's important to untangle these two concepts: being alone and being lonely. While there's some overlap between them, they're completely different concepts. Maybe you're a person who basks in solitude. You're not antisocial, friendless, or loveless. You're just quite content with alone time. You look forward to it. That's simply being alone, not being lonely.

On the other hand, maybe you're surrounded by family and friends but not relating beyond a surface level, which has you feeling empty and disconnected. Or maybe being alone just leaves you sad and longing for company. That's loneliness.

Short-term tips to get you started

These tips are aimed at helping you get the ball rolling. They might not transform your life overnight, but they can help you get more comfortable with being alone.

Some of them may be exactly what you needed to hear. Others may not make sense to you. Use them as stepping-stones. Add to them and shape them along the way to suit your lifestyle and personality.

1. **Avoid comparing yourself to others.**

This is easier said than done, but try to avoid comparing your social life to anyone else's. It's not the number of friends you have or the frequency of your social outings that matters. It's what works for you.

Remember, you have no way of knowing if someone with many friends and a stuffed social calendar is happy.

2. **Take a step back from social media.**

Social media isn't inherently bad or problematic, but if scrolling through your feeds makes you feel left out and stresses, take a few steps back. That feed doesn't tell the whole story. Not by a long shot.

You have no idea if those people are truly happy or just giving the impression that they are. Either way, it's no reflection on you. So, take a deep breath and put it in perspective.

Perform a test run and ban yourself from social media for 48 hours. If that makes a difference, try giving yourself a daily limit of 10 to 15 minutes and stick to it.

Don't be afraid to ask for help.

Sometimes, all the self-care, exercise, and gratitude lists in the world aren't enough to shake feelings of sadness or loneliness.

Consider reaching out to a therapist if:

- You're overly <u>stressed</u> and finding it difficult to cope.

- You have <u>symptoms of anxiety</u>.

- You have <u>symptoms of depression</u>.

You don't have to wait for a crisis point to get into <u>therapy</u>. Simply wanting to get better and spending time alone is a perfectly good reason to make an appointment.

Chapter 9:

Happy People Take Care of Themselves

I frequently hear the word "selfish" tossed about in coaching, often with a negative connotation. Someone feels bad that they were selfish or that someone else was selfish, and it was offensive. Selfishness – the lack of considering others or only being concerned with your advantage – can be a great weakness. The ability to put others' needs in front of your own is an important life skill that you need to be able to do without resentment, even when it's completely inconvenient and a sacrifice.

However, I would argue that the motivation behind that decision should be self-serving. In most cases, being selfish is just a matter of perspective, critical to happiness and self-evolution.

Let me explain…

First, let's talk about why it is so important to be selfish. As author <u>Brené Brown</u> has discovered in her research on wholehearted living, loving yourself more than you love others is the first and most critical step to seeking happiness and fulfillment.

She says it is impossible to love anyone more than you love yourself. Taking care of yourself is the pathway to fulfillment and high performance in work and life. And, just as importantly, it's a gift to others.

When your needs are met, and you feel good about yourself, it's easier to elevate other people's needs in front of your own. It's easy to be a giver when your cup is full. When you feel half-full or empty, it's harder to give. You inherently feel people should be giving more to you or others, so you don't have to give so much or feel you need to preserve more for yourself.

Here are the two common derailments that can prevent you from finding fulfillment:

1. Giving too much

When people give too much - continually put other people's needs ahead of their own - builds resentment and takes away from their ability to take care of themselves. When their time is so focused on others, they don't have any time left for themselves. I find people do this when they are uncomfortable asking for their needs, speaking up about issues, or delegating responsibilities. Often they hide these weaknesses by focusing on other people, so they don't have to focus on themselves. This not only leads to feeling unfulfilled but becomes a burden on others who feel they need to take care of the "giver."

2. Taking too much time for ourselves

On the opposite end of the spectrum, some people take too much time for themselves, mistakenly thinking it will lead to fulfillment. They do not "give" enough, and it usually makes them feel worse, disengaging them from relationships and putting them on a treadmill of trying to do something that will finally make them feel good. In these cases, they are usually working on the wrong issues. The places where they are investing their time do not give them meaning.

Chapter 10:

Make Your Life Better By Saying

'Thank You'

We are an ungrateful species. We are not grateful enough for what we have on our plates or for what someone else does for it. Even if we are on the receiving end of it, we don't appreciate it much.

We think that the word 'Thank you should be reserved for a very special moment. We treat it as if it is a very posh word and can't be used in many instances. But the reality is that we are not grateful enough to have the courage to thank more than we are doing right now.

You are not losing anything and it certainly doesn't affect your image in others' eyes. It surely helps to get things done more easily and quickly if you were to thank more often. It would help you get a better place in others' judgment of you and it would help you fit in with anyone.

Let's say you were to receive congrats for any of your achievements from any of your colleagues. Would it be rude if you weren't to return the compliment with a simple 'Thank You'?

Wouldn't you be called an egotistical person for not even appreciating the other with a simple compliment?

What if you were to say 'Thank You' for even the smallest of virtues happening to you? You would be praised for your gratitude towards others and you would be celebrated even more for even your smallest achievements.

You not only have to thank the people around you, but you should also thank god or your luck or your life for every moment that led you to this day.

Thank you for the hard times that made you appreciate the good times. Thank you for the lessons that you needed for you personal development. Thank you for a healthy life. Thank you for all the energies that drive me. Thank you for the drive. Thank you for the confidence. Thank you for my spirit. Thank you for the courage to keep me going through the hard times. Thank you for everything that we take for granted.

You should thank the people in your life that make your life worth living for. Thank them more than often because they have done a lot for you and also thank them for everything they will do for you in the future.

It won't hurt you to be grateful to others and it won't make anyone want you less. It will only increase your importance in others' life and them wanting to do more for you.

Take some time out of your life every day and just run your whole day like a flashback. Concentrate on the moments of respect and kindness that you received from anyone. Take some time out the next day and just go and thank them all. You would be surprised by what you receive from them, and what it makes you feel for yourself. Your trust in humanity will be immortal with this simple habit!

Chapter 11:

Happy People Consciously Nurture A Growth Mindset

"Without continual growth and progress, such words as improvement, achievement, and success have no meaning." – Benjamin Franklin

Learning is perceived and generally acknowledged by those of us who have gone through primary and university tutoring. We were routinely encircled by people who energized and upheld our developments. Groundbreaking thoughts and change were anticipated from us; the sky was the limit!! However, shouldn't something be said about once we got into the work environment? For some, we subsided into the everyday daily practice, getting it done, uninformed of the cost that our agreeable, monotonous, continuous tasks appeared to have on our own and expert development.

Do you hear employees saying, "I don't get how this venture's development works" or "I'm awful at giving introductions. If it's not too much trouble, let another person do it." If this is the case, reconsideration of your group's growth mindset might be in order. They are working under a "fixed mentality." According to an examination concentrate via Carol Dweck of Stanford University, a fixed attitude happens when individuals accept fixed qualities that can't change. These individuals archive abilities instead of attempting to foster them. On the other hand, a development attitude accepts that knowledge can develop with time and experience. When individuals accept they can add to their learning, they understand exertion affects their prosperity.

You can attempt to battle a fixed attitude and energize a sound growth mindset by rehearsing the following:

Recognize fixed mindset patterns

To begin with, would you say you are ready to precisely recognize and uncover the negative quirks coming about because of a fixed mentality? Normal practices of these individuals incorporate the individuals who keep away from challenges, surrender effectively, consider there to be as achieving nothing, overlook and keep away from negative criticism, need heading in their objectives, and carry on when feeling undermined by other people who make progress. These are normal signs that employees are battling to see their part in supporting the new turn of events.

Energize feedback over praise

Commendation feels better. We like to feel approved in our qualities and are content to let it be the point at which we get acclaim over achieved work—employees to request input despite the result. There are consistent approaches to improve and create. Lead your group to request tips and innovative manners by which they can move toward new situations.

Pinpoint skills and limitations

Take time out from the ordinary daily schedule to pinpoint your workers' qualities and shortcomings will give an unmistakable beginning stage to an initiative in realizing where holes exist. Have workers independently take strength evaluations and meet with them to go over outcomes. Some may feel compromised and cautious while going over shortcomings, yet having a direct discussion on the finding will prompt better anticipation and recuperating.

Chapter 12:

To Make Big Gains, Avoid Tiny Losses

Life is a process of adding and subtracting. We add the things that make us better and make life easier. We put aside the things that prove to be a pebble in the shoe.

There is a flaw in human effort and our concept for success. We think that we can achieve more if we focus harder on getting better. We think that if we are not getting worse, we are on the right track. But I can assure you, we are heavily mistaken.

The more we focus on bigger gains, the more we overlook the small things we stop caring about. We give up on relations, hobbies, ethics, love, and the million other losses that we don't measure on the same scale.

We can achieve the same amount of things, the same scale of success, and still, be the better person that we want to be. But we don't need to not work on the smaller details of this successful journey.

Let's say you have achieved it all and now you look back a decade or two. Do you think you won't regret the things that could have been saved in this whole process? But you chose not to or didn't care enough for them, and now you are rich in the pocket but poor in every other sense.

They say money can buy you anything, but it can never buy you happiness. You can have all the money in the world but you can't make sure if you won't ever have any regret.

We all are a creator. We make things, sometimes for ourselves and sometimes for people around us. Sometimes we make things better for us that then prove to be good for someone else as well. But also do things in a way that doesn't affect anyone else in a bad way. At least not deliberately.

Bad things happen, but most of the time we are the reason for them to happen in the first place. We are so devoted to the greater good that we neglect the small things we lose in the process. Check it with yourself, if you are so devoted to being a better person than you were yesterday, and you have achieved more than yesterday. Then why do you still repeat the small mistakes and take the small losses?

You have to understand the concept of losses over gains. If you invest some money into something, and you are at a small loss every other day, then you can't justify the big profits you might gain some days later.

It is the constant concern to keep away from the small misfortunes or mistakes that might leave you into yet another breakdown. If you truly want to be a free and successful person, you need to have confidence in whatever you do will certainly give you more and more and it won't come at the cost of a single thing. Take the mantra, reduce your losses and your gains will gain volumes in no time.

Chapter 13:

How To Become A Morning Person

Our natural sleep/wake cycles are known as our circadian rhythm, and they can vary a lot from person to person. People fall into different groups, or chronotypes, depending on whether they feel most awake and alert in the morning, in the evening or somewhere in between.

No chronotype is inherently better or worse than another. There's nothing wrong with staying up late and sleeping in. "If that schedule fits with your lifestyle and your obligations, it's not necessary to change it."

The trouble comes when your late bedtime clashes with your early morning obligations. If you're regularly getting less than the recommended seven to nine hours of sleep a night, your health and well-being can suffer.

Unfortunately, we can't pick our chronotypes. Genetics plays a part in whether you identify as a night owl or a morning lark. Still, your habits and behaviours can reinforce those natural tendencies. And those habits aren't set in stone. "By making behavioural changes, you may be able to shift your sleep schedule preferences,"

How to reset your circadian rhythm? How, exactly, do you become more of a morning person?

Shift your bedtime: Count back from the time your alarm rings, aiming for a total of seven to nine hours a night. That will be your target bedtime — eventually. If you're used to turning in well after midnight, willing yourself to suddenly fall asleep at 10:00 p.m. is sure to backfire.

Aim to go to bed 15 or 20 minutes earlier than usual for a few days. Then push it back another 15 minutes for several more days. "It's important to adjust your sleep time gradually," she says.

Make it routine: A quiet bedtime routine is key to helping you fall asleep earlier. At least an hour before lights out, dim the lights and power down your electronics. Find something soothing to do, like taking a warm bath, reading a book or listening to a (not-too-stimulating) podcast. "Give yourself time to wind down and prepare your mind for bed."

Lighten up: "Our circadian rhythms are responsive to light and dark," Exposure to bright light first thing in the morning helps you feel more alert and also helps shift your internal rhythm toward an earlier wake time.

Natural light is the best, so get outside or open your bedroom window. If you can't get outside or your room is natural light-deprived, try a light therapy lamp that mimics the spectrum of natural light.

Make mornings more pleasant: Try to schedule something to look forward to in the morning so that getting up feels like less of a slog. Perhaps a hot cup of coffee, sipped in silence, and the daily crossword puzzle. Knowing that something pleasant awaits can help you take that first, painful step out of bed.

Move your alarm clock: Hitting snooze is all too tempting, so remove that option. Try putting your alarm clock across the room, so you have to get up to turn it off.

Some apps make it even harder to sleep in, by forcing you to engage in mentally stimulating activities like solving a puzzle to stop the beeping. "Do whatever works to keep you from hitting snooze,"

Chapter 14:

9 Tips To Reduce Stress

Stress and anxiety are common experiences for most people. In fact, 70% of adults in the United States say they feel stress or anxiety daily. Here are 16 simple ways to relieve stress and anxiety.

1. Exercise

Exercise is one of the most important things you can do to combat stress. It might seem contradictory, but putting physical stress on your body through exercise can relieve mental stress. The benefits are strongest when you exercise regularly. People who exercise regularly are less likely to experience anxiety than those who don't exercise. Activities such as walking or jogging that involve repetitive movements of large muscle groups can be particularly stress relieving.

2. Consider supplements

Several supplements promote stress and anxiety reduction. Here is a brief overview of some of the most common ones:

Lemon balm: Lemon balm is a member of the mint family that has been studied for its anti-anxiety effects.

Omega-3 fatty acids: One study showed that medical students who received omega-3 supplements experienced a 20% reduction in anxiety symptoms.

Ashwagandha: Ashwagandha is an herb used in Ayurvedic medicine to treat stress and anxiety. Several studies suggest that it's effective.

Green tea: Green tea contains many polyphenol antioxidants which provide health benefits. It may lower stress and anxiety by increasing serotonin levels.

Valerian: Valerian root is a popular sleep aid due to its tranquilizing effect. It contains valerenic acid, which alters gamma-aminobutyric acid (GABA) receptors to lower anxiety.

Some supplements can interact with medications or have side effects, so you may want to consult with a doctor if you have a medical condition.

3. Light a candle

Using essential oils or burning a scented candle may help reduce your feelings of stress and anxiety.

Some scents are especially soothing. Here are some of the most calming scents:

- Lavender
- Rose
- Vetiver
- Bergamot
- Roman chamomile
- Neroli
- Frankincense
- Orange or orange blossom
- Geranium

Using scents to treat your mood is called aromatherapy. Several studies show that aromatherapy can decrease anxiety and improve sleep.

4. Reduce your caffeine intake

Caffeine is a stimulant found in coffee, tea, chocolate and energy drinks. High doses can increase anxiety. People have different thresholds for how much caffeine they can tolerate. If you notice that caffeine makes you jittery or anxious, consider cutting back. Although many studies show that coffee can be healthy in moderation, it's not for everyone. In general, five or fewer cups per day is considered a moderate amount.

5. Write it down

One way to handle stress is to write things down. While recording what you're stressed about is one approach, another is jotting down what you're grateful for. Gratitude may help relieve stress and anxiety by focusing your thoughts on what's positive in your life.

6. Chew gum

For a super easy and quick stress reliever, try chewing a stick of gum. One study showed that people who chewed gum had a greater sense of wellbeing and lower stress. One possible explanation is that chewing gum causes brain waves similar to those of relaxed people. Another is that chewing gum promotes blood flow to your brain. Additionally, one recent study found that stress relief was greatest when people chewed more strongly.

7. Spend time with friends and family

Social support from friends and family can help you get through stressful times. Being part of a friend network gives you a sense of belonging and self-worth, which can help you in tough times. One study found that for women in particular, spending time with friends and children helps release oxytocin, a natural stress reliever. This effect is called "tend and befriend," and is the opposite of the fight-or-flight response. Keep in mind that both men and women benefit from friendship. Another study found that men and women with the fewest social connections were more likely to suffer from depression and anxiety.

8. Laugh

It's hard to feel anxious when you're laughing. It's good for your health, and there are a few ways it may help relieve stress: Relieving your stress response. Relieving tension by relaxing your muscles.

In the long term, laughter can also help improve your immune system and mood. A study among people with cancer found that people in the laughter intervention group experienced more stress relief than those who were simply distracted. Try watching a funny TV show or hanging out with friends who make you laugh.

9. Learn to say no

Try not to take on more than you can handle. Saying no is one way to control your stressors.

Chapter 15:

Resist Temptations For Success

We all have hopes and dreams. We have a rough sketch of what we want to become and what we want to achieve. Most of us have good intentions for those things too.

But the reality is that process of achieving those things isn't always as simple as we all anticipate. It is all mixed up with all these temptations that are equally alluring and want us to give up everything else for just a moment and enjoy what we are about to indulge in.

You see if you were to make a milestone for a week where you were to lose a pound of weight with rigorous cardio and hours of strict training followed by a strict diet plan. You can't say you won't be tempted by the smell of fries and fried chicken whenever you walk past one.

Surely you would be OK, only if you resisted it and kept walking your way. But if you were to pick up one piece and put it in your mouth, you just destroyed the whole mantra of self-control and self-discipline.

Self-discipline is not just putting your life on track and following a timetable. Self-discipline is not punishing yourself for any mistake. Self-discipline is following a course of actions that will take you to your ultimate goal.

We all are susceptible to weaknesses. We often end up acting against the things and goals that we value the most.

Temptations are nature's way of testing us. It is a test to evaluate our core values and our integrity. It is a litmus test to pick the leaders out of a faction. Temptations are a way of self-analyzing ourselves whether we are worthy enough or are we still distracted with all the shiny things lying around.

It is easy to get a good grade with a little help from here and there. It is easy to follow someone else's path rather than carving our own. It is easier to fake some lab results to be enrolled into a team of representatives.

But when we get the chance to do those things in real life without any outside help on an open stage where the world is judging us, we cannot get ourselves to do any of those things because we cheated n the first place and never engaged the creative factory of our mind.

So how should you approach this problem? It is a simple step-by-step process.

Start by removing the temptations. Check for any loopholes in your environment and kick them out to keep them away long enough till you are more in control.

Next, you need to take some time to think about your way of thinking as an unbiased and nonhuman object. Try to find the flaws and reinvent them to disengage any magnets in your personality that keep attracting you to those temptations.

Last but not the least, put a zipper on your pocket and control your spending habits and you will get away from any unnecessary temptation leading you to a better successful life!

Chapter 16:

Develop Mental Toughness In The Face of Adversity

The drawback of this technological revolution that we live in is that we have created a weaker generation, a weaker society. We need everything to be perfect, to be exactly the way we want it to be.

We can't bear a single change in our routines. We can't handle a single harmless task that might test us in any way possible. We can't forgive anyone's mistake but we want all our blunders to be erased.

We can't handle the fact that life is always a step ahead of us. And if something bad happens, we try to mask it. We never try to actually deal with the problems, rather keep them at bay as long as we can.

We are so afraid of trying the do the things that would matter, but we become the wisest when we mock or advise someone else.

We are never truly prepared for the hard times. We are always in a constant fight with our own minds, neglecting reality and creating a false scenario where everything is alright. It is not Alright!

We are living in a time where everyone is in search of greatness. There are more and more people coming into this world every day and the competition is getting harder than it ever was. The day will come when we would have to fight for even the basic necessities of life.

The day might come when we will fail at almost everything we are doing right now. What will we do then?

Life gives us second chances, but those chances require us to be stronger. Those chances want us to first create some chances beforehand before we go forward with the grand scheme.

Chances present themselves to the people who are in the constant struggle to live every minute as if it were their last.

If someone was to ask you to join them for a morning run, you might be enthusiastic for one day. You will wake up at five in the morning, gear up, and go for 10 miles for the first day. On the second day, you will go for it again. A week later you will take a break for a day. A month later you might get a treadmill because you feel more comfortable running in your home rather than going out in the cold mornings. But eventually, you will stop doing it.

All of this is because you are not ready to get out of your comfort zone or not ready to commit for long enough to achieve what you started for.

Learn to say 'No' to 'No'. The day you start saying no to everything that will keep you in your warm cozy bed, is the day you will finally realize what you will achieve that day.

Life will always be hard on you, but you can join the league of successful beings if you stay true to your cause and keep pushing and digging till you finally find the gem of your choice.

Chapter 17:

Stop Wasting Time on the Details and Commit to the Fundamentals

Time runs on a treadmill that has no apparent switch. We have a timeline on this planet and it will come to an end sooner or later. It would be sooner than we think, that is for sure!

But what we put in, to live what time we have to make it matter for if it were our last second, is a concept I'll try to endorse here.

You see, we all live our lives as if no one is more sincere and dedicated than we are. We put in all the hours and we put in all the energy but we can't guarantee anything, can we?

It is never about how hardworking you are. It is never about the rules and the intricacies of things we follow. It is never about the hours we put in, but what we put into the hours!

This is not as simple as it may sound. We, humans, have a common flaw as an intelligent species. It is an adherent flaw in our upbringing and the norms that we follow.

We don't know what is more important, is it the plane or the pilot? We have what we call an instinctive nature that draws us to conclusions and things that will influence us to ultimately find our purpose, but in that process of finding one, we lose focus of what we have at hand right now!

We are working straight hours for things that have secondary importance in our lives and sometimes can be discouraging. We are working so hard on things that have least to no contribution to our happiness and success but we are still going on around them foolishly.

Not everything is meant to be done and not everything is meant to bring meaning to the spice of life. But we still do it because we are naive and shallow.

We need to learn what are the fundamentals of living a successful life.

You don't have a single aspect of your life to take care of. You can't dedicate the majority of your time and attention to fixing only one thing when there are a lot more and lot better things to take care of.

You don't need to avoid the bigger and bolder realities just because you are afraid you might fail and fall. You surely can and you surely will. You only have to keep trying and you will eventually set things straight.

Set your priorities in the right direction. You don't need a fancy logo for your business if you haven't had a single paying customer yet. You can't have a better grade if you haven't done any of the term work. You can't expect to be paid a full wager if you have dozens of chores still pending for the next day.

The details are useless if you haven't had the fundamentals done yet. The final formula has no meaning if you had the basic equation wrong. So follow the process and the process will lead you to the final viewpoint!

Chapter 18:

Mastering One Thing At A Time

I don't think anyone needs any explanation for the phrase, "Jack of all trades, Master of none". If you are one of those people who still can't get a grasp of this simple yet effective phenomenon, you seriously need to revisit your approach to life.

No one can be a true master. It's only a title for comparison. Mastering even one thing can be a task that can take decades. And once you become one, you can't guarantee you would remain the only person eligible for the title.

Yes, you would argue that you want to perfect everything because you want a better life and don't want any acknowledgment or applause. And I know it is well justified, but you need to focus on the bigger things.

Acknowledgment is important. It gives us the confidence to do more. But satisfying others for them to satisfy you is a stupid reason to pursue something. There is a lot of big fish out there for you to go and hunt.

You can go running around all day fetching small motives and goals, which would never profit you in the long run of life. Bigger chances always lie around us, but we are always too distracted to wait and get a good grasp of just one.

Instead of holding onto the one major thing, we cling to countless small ones and end up getting a little bit of everything. But we want everything and a lot of it, as our nature dictates us.

But the truth is simple yet harsh, "You can't always get what you want". You will never be able to get a hold of everything. But you can be good at just one thing and then try to make up the ladder with other singular things, goals, desires, wishes. And who knows, they might eventually get granted one by one.

We spend our life chasing so many things that we eventually get to a point where we are so exhausted that nothing encourages us and we end up giving away all the hard work that we put in.

But life isn't always about giving up on everything else just for the sake of one thing. This misconception is common for everyone that if I go for one goal only, I might not get another chance for the others I had dreamt of.

You need to set your priorities straight. If you have a long-term goal, you need to go for the basics first and gradually climb up the ladder for the ultimate ideal for success.

But consistency and dedication are the traits that once you develop will always help you master everything that you ever come across till your last day on this planet.

Learn to say no to everything that gets in between you and your task at hand. Set your goals for the day and execute everything one by one. Don't leave anything half done, rather give every task your whole effort and your every new venture will see the dawn.

Chapter 19:

Do You Know What You Want?

Do you know who you are? Do you know what you are? Do you know what you want to become? Do you have any idea what you might become?

Every sane human has asked these questions to themselves multiple times in their lives. We have a specific trait of always finding the right answers to everything. We humans always try to find the meaning behind everything.

It's in our built-in nature to question everything around us. Yet we are here in this modern era of technology and resources and we don't have a sense of purpose. We don't have a true set of goals. We don't give enough importance to our future to take a second and make a long-term plan for longer gains.

The fault in our thinking is that we don't have a strict model of attention. We have too many distractions in our lives to spare a moment to clear our minds.

The other thing that makes us confused or ignorant is the fact that people have a way of leading us into thinking things that are not ours to start with.

Society has made these norms that have absolutely nothing to do with anyone except that these were someone's experience when they were once at our stage. We are dictated on things that are not ours to achieve but only a mere image of what others want us to achieve or don't.

No one has the right to tell you anything. No one has a right to say anything to you except if they are advising or reminding you of the worst. But to inflict a scenario with such surety that it will eventually happen to you because you have a fault that many others had before you is the most superstitious and illogical thing to do on any planet let alone Earth.
No one knows what the future holds for anyone. No one can guarantee even the next breath that they take. So why put yourself under someone else's spell of disappointment? Why do you feel the need to satisfy every person's whim? Why do you feel content with everyone around you getting their ways?

You always know in your heart, deep down in some corner what you want. You will always know what you need to be fulfilled. You will always find an inspiration within yourself to go and pursue that thing. What you need are some self-confidence and some self-motivation. You need to give yourself some time to straighten up your thoughts and you will eventually get the BOLD statement stating 'This is what I want'.

You don't need to shut everyone around you. You just need to fix your priorities and you will get a vivid image of what things are and what they can become.

There is no constraint of age or gender to achieving anything. These are just mental and emotional hurdles that we have imposed on our whole race throughout our history.

Just remember. When you know what you want, and you want it bad enough to give away everything for that, you will someday find a way to finally get it.

Chapter 20:

10 Habits That Can Ruin Your Day

Habits are the building blocks of our day. No matter how you spin it, either way, every detail matters.

The little actionable habits eventually sets you up to a either having a fulfilling day, or one that you have just totally wasted away. Nothing is as bad as destructive habits as they sabotage your daily productivity. Slowly, you slip further and further until it's too late when you've realized the damage that they have done to your life.

Bad habits are insidious! They drag down your life, lowers down your levels of accuracy, and make your performance less creative and stifling. It is essential, not only for productivity, to gain control of your bad habits. AS Grenville Kleiser once noted, "Constant self-discipline and self-control help you develop greatness of character." Nonetheless, it is important to stop and ask: what do you need today to get rid of or change? Sure, you can add or adjust new skills into your daily life.

Below are ten persistent habits that can ruin your day's success and productivity.

1. Hitting The Snooze Button.

Your mind, while you sleep, moves through a comprehensive series of cycles, the last one alerting you to wake up. While you crave for ten more minutes of sleep as the alarm goes off, what do you do? You whacked the snooze button. We're all guilty of this! If you don't suck it up, rip off the cover and start your morning, the rest of your day will be flawed. How do you expect your day to be strong once you don't start it off strong? You will feel far more optimistic, strong and fully prepared when you wake up without hitting the snooze button. So avoid the snooze button at any cost if you want a productive day ahead!

2. Wasting Your "Getting Ready" Hours.

You might need to reconsider the scrolling of Instagram and Facebook or the inane program you put on behind the scenes while preparing. These things have a time and place to partake in them – for example when you've accomplished your day's work and need some time to unwind and relax; however the time isn't now. Your morning schedule ought to be an interaction that prepares and energizes you for the day ahead. The objective is to accomplish something that animates your mind within the first hour of being conscious, so you can be more inventive, invigorated, gainful, and connected with all through the entire day! Avoiding this sweeps you away from normalizing the worst habit you might have: distraction. Instead, give yourself a chance to breathe the fine morning, anticipate the day's wonder and be thankful for whatever you have.

3. Failing To Prioritize Your Breakfast.

Energizing your day is essential if you wish for a very productive day. Energizing your body system requires that you prioritize eating your breakfast. However, the contents of your breakfast must entail something that will ensure that your day is not slowed down by noon. This means a blend of high - fiber foods such as proteins and healthy must be incorporated. Avoid taking too many sugars and heavy starches. The goal is to satiate and energize your body for the day.

4. Ruminating on the Problems of Yesterday And Negativity.

Don't take yesterday's problems to your new day if you want to start your day off right. If the day before you had difficult meetings and talks and you woke up ruminating about your horrific experiences, leave that negativity at your doorway. Moreover, if the problem you are lamenting about have been solved, then you shouldn't dwell on the past. Research suggests that we usually encounter more positive than negative events in a day. Still, often your mind concentrates on the negative due to a subconscious distortion called the negative distortion. By choosing not to focus on negative events and thinking about what's going well, you can learn to take advantage of the strength of the positive events around us. Raising negativity only increases stress. Let go of it and get on without it!

5. Leaving Your Day To Randomness.

Do not let stuff just simply happen to you; do it. Failure to create a structured day leads to a totally random day. A random day lacking direction, focus, and efficiency. Distractions will also creep into your day more readily because you have allowed randomness to happen to you. Instead, have a clear and precise list of what you need to focus for the day. This serves as a framework and a boundary for you to work within. Another thing you should consider is to spend your first 90 minutes on the most thoughtful and important task for the day. This allows you to know the big things out right at the beginning, reducing your cognitive burden for the rest of the day.

6. Becoming Involved With the Overview.

How frequently have you woken up, and before you can stretch and grin, you groan pretty much all the have-to for now and the fragmented musts from yesterday? This unhealthy habit will ruin your great day ahead. Know and understand these are simply contemplations. You can decide to recalibrate by pondering all you must be thankful for and searching for the splendid focuses in your day. Shift thinking, and you'll begin the day empowered.

7. Overscheduling and Over-Engagement.

People tend to underestimate how long things take with so many things to do. This habit of overscheduling and over-engagement can quickly lead to burn out. Always ensure that you permit extra time and energy for the unforeseen. Take regular breaks and don't overcommit to other people. This gives you more freedom for yourself and you won't be running the risk of letting others down by not turning up. Try not to overestimate what you can complete, so you won't feel like a disappointment. Be sensible and practical with your scheduling. Unexpectedly and eventually, you'll complete more.

8. Postponing or Discarding the Tough Tasks.

We have a restricted measure of mental energy, and as we exhaust this energy, our dynamic and efficiency decrease quickly. This is called decision exhaustion. Running the bad habit of postponing and disregarding the tough tasks will trigger this reaction in us. At the point when you put off extreme assignments till late in the day because they're scary, you deplete more and more of your mental resources. To beat choice weariness, you should handle complex assignments toward the beginning of the day when your brain is new.

9. Failure To Prioritize Your Self-Care.

Work, family commitments, and generally talking of the general obligations give almost everyone an awesome excuse to let your self-care rehearses pass by the wayside. Achievement-oriented minds of individuals see how basic self-care is to their expert achievement. Invest energy doing things that bring you delight and backing your psychological and actual wellbeing. "Success" doesn't exclusively apply to your finances or expert accomplishments.

10. Waiting for the Easier Way Out / Waiting for the Perfect Hack of Your Life.

The most noticeably awful everyday habit is trusting that things will occur and for a chance to thump at your entryway. As such, you become an inactive onlooker, not a proactive part of your own life. Once in a while, it shows itself as the quest for simple little-known techniques. Rather than getting down to work, ineffective individuals search how to take care of job quicker for quite a long time. Try not to begin with a #lifehack search on the internet unless it really does improve your productivity without sacrificing the necessary steps you need to take each day to achieve holistic success.

✓ Merging It All Together

A portion of these habits may appear to be minor, yet they add up. Most amount to an individual decision between immediate pleasures and enduring ones. The most exceedingly awful propensity is forgetting about what matters to you. Always remember that you are just one habit away from changing you life forever.

Chapter 21:

8 Ways To Turn Stress Into Strength

We tend to think of stress as all bad, but it doesn't have to be. Without stress, we might feel less motivated, and if we're pushing our life forward, getting things done and achieving our goals, stress will always be part of that. Stress is a fixed and natural part of our lives so, instead of trying to fight it or get rid of it, we need to make stress work for us by learning how to manage it better. Here are 10 ways you can manage your stress and make it work for you

1.Build a 'stress wall'

During stressful periods, you might feel bombarded by stressful thoughts that trigger anxiety. When a thought comes, try using active imagination to combat it. Imagine the worry bouncing off a big impenetrable wall in your mind and floating away from your immediate attention. Keep that wall up until you're ready to deal with the problem, and imagine all the further stressful thoughts continuing to bounce off it. When you stop allowing stressful thoughts to permeate your mind, you'll be able to manage stress a lot more effectively.

You don't have to imagine a wall - you can choose any thought metaphor that suits you. You might prefer to imagine your thoughts as birds landing on a tree and you make them fly away again or putting your thoughts into a box and closing the lid.

2. Stop living in the world of what if

When we're stressed, we live in the world of what if.

What if this happens?... What if I can't do that?... What if I make a fool out of myself?

Most of these worrying thoughts never happen, and they're only getting in your way. Try to stop living in the world of what if and start living in the land of the real. So what if something doesn't go quite right? You've just learned something new, and there is always value in that. Don't be afraid to take a chance.

3. Focus on positive people

Where your lifestyle allows it, try to spend more time with people who will have a positive influence on your wellbeing. This doesn't necessarily mean people who don't get as stressed as you - in fact someone who is going through the same emotions as you could act as a buddy and you could help each other to be more productive with your stress management.

4. Learn to let go

If you have a heavy workload or money/relationship worries, it makes you feel out of control. Feeling out of control causes stress. The more we fight to control a situation the more stressed it makes us. Accept that it's not possible to control every situation in life. Unclench your fists, lower your shoulders and stop screwing up your face. Take a breath and let it go - for instant stress relief.

5. Set a deadline

Parkinson's law says "work expands so as to fill the time available for its completion". In other words, if you set a deadline you're more likely to get a task done within that timescale. By not having a deadline, you're risking living a life filled with unfinished business. That's only going to lead to one thing: stress! Set a deadline on every task that comes up in your life and watch how much more you get done.

6. Be present and mindful

Stress is usually related to our past and future – worrying about what we've done and what we need to do. Take a second to appreciate this moment, right now. The more often you can live in the present the less stressed you're going to be. The past is over, and the future hasn't happened yet. Are they really worth all that worry?

7. Focus on what you want

Whatever you focus on, and put more energy into, you're going to get more of it in your life. Focus on being stressed, and there are no prizes for guessing what you'll get in return. Try focusing on what it is you want, and you'll naturally gravitate in that direction. Write down your targets and goals right now, and make those your focus.

8. Be grateful

Lack of gratitude breeds stressful thoughts and feelings. Practice being grateful for what you have, rather than worrying about what you don't have. Think about five things you can be grateful for right now. Take five every day and practice being more grateful.

You should also sometimes feel grateful for your feelings of stress as, without them, feeling relaxed wouldn't be as satisfying.

Chapter 22:

10 Habits of Ariana Grande

You may remember Ariana Grande from her early days as Cat Valentine on the Nickelodeon sitcoms "Victorious" and her show "Sam and Cat," as well as her music, including her latest album, "Positions." Her career took off after she decided to pursue music. She creates music that combines pop, Electronica, and R&b music.

Ariana Grande is an American singer and actress with over 126 awards in her music career. She is also an activist who has constantly been speaking out in support of women and LGBT rights. Her superpowers, both on and off stage, have landed her on time's list of the world's most influential people.

Although she is well known for her powerful vocals, there is way lot more to her than you know. Here are 10 Ariana Grande habits that might intrigue you.

1. She Puts Her Ego Aside

It's easy to let your ego kick in when the world is constantly talking about you. But for Ariana Grande, her ego and what she loves doing can't mingle as it can drag her work, which she finds unacceptable.

When does your ego get in the way of your masterpiece? Are you spending more time focusing on other people's work or on what other people have to say? Take a cue from Ariana Grande.

2. She Stands Her Ground

As a feminist, Ariana does not let anyone or anything get in her way, but she does so professionally. Possibly Grande explains it best when she encourages others to be themselves rather than living up to expectations. You can be gorgeous and clever, nice and goofy while strong and invincible as well as simultaneously sexual and entertaining.

3. She Maintains a Healthy Environment

Ariana Grande has held fast to her roots by surrounding herself with health and love. Her circle of friends and family are people she grew up with within Boca Raton. Keeping close to people that matter more in her life help her stay grounded and sane.

Your surrounding will influence your habits and behaviour towards improving and moving quickly.

4. She Does Her Own Thing

There are certain steps that everyone has taken when advancing through the ranks of whichever industry they chose. Like you start here and work your way up, doing this first, then that.

Just because there is a historical record of how things were doesn't mean they have to stay that way. Grande is a beautiful example of this: her dream was to be a singer, but she wanted to release songs in the way that a rapper does.

5. Continues Improving

Do you have a plan to improve? It would be ideal if you monitored your habits daily to ensure that you are consistently showing up and making modest improvements to your life. Ariana Grande surpassed her heavy net worth by improving and staying on top of her game. From "victorious" to creating her show "Sam and Cat" to building an empire through her music career.

6. She Takes Care of Her Emotional Wellbeing

If Grande's hit song "thank u, next" doesn't express her dating review, consider this: she guards her mental space. She constantly reminds her fans how important it is to protect their mental health and peace. Ground, exhaust, and conserve your mental health with the right energy.

7. She Makes Her Dreams Come True

Just like Ariana, manifest it! Ask any new life guru, astrology, or life coach, and they'll insist on manifestation. This is the where you envision, believe and trust that the things you desire will fall into place.

8. Simplicity Is Her Fineness

Looking like Ariana Grande may be your dream and a challenge too. When it comes to self-care, simplicity characterizes her. Ariana maintains a vegan diet, takes regular strolls, and naps enough to keep her health intact.

9. Don't Let Haters Get Your Cool

Ariana got blamed for her Ex-boyfriend, Mac Miller death, and aftermath of Manchester bombing. Despite these, she managed to ace her record-breaking album "sweeter" to honour the lives lost during the bombing.

10. Looks Don't Define You

Occasionally, Ariana reminds her fans not to allow their looks or weight define who they really are. No one is perfect, just be true to your sweet self.

Conclusion

Ariana is a true sweetheart, and above all, she seems to be growing much stronger despite all the backlash she receives publicly. Even though you don't agree with all her actions, there is definitely something to grasps from her habits.

Chapter 23:

Live A Long, Important Life

Do you think you are more capable to deal with the failure or the regret of not trying at all?

Are you living the life you want or the life everyone else wants for you?

Would you feel good spending your time on entertainment that might not last for long? Or would you feel good feeling like you are growing and have a better self of you to look at in the mirror?

Similarly, would like to live in the present or would you love to work for a better future?

Do you want money to dictate your life or do you want money to follow you where ever you go?

Would you prefer being tired or being broke?

Do you want to spend the rest of your life in this place where you and your parents were born? Or do you won't go around the world and find new possibilities in even the most remote places?

Would you rather risk it all or play it safe?

We are often presented with all these questions in our lifetime. Most people take these questions as a way to enter into your adulthood. The answers to these questions are meant to show you the actual meaning of life.

So what is Life? Life is not your parents, your work, your friends, your events, and your functions. It's within you and around you.

You should learn to live your life to the fullest. You should love to live your life for as long as you can with a happy body and a healthy mind.

A happy and healthy body and mind are important. Because you can only feel secure on a stable platform. You can only wish to stand on a platform where you know you can stay put for a long time.

There is nothing wrong with working eight or nine hours in your daily life. It's not unhealthy or anything. Working is what gives our life a purpose. Working is what keeps us active, moving, and motivated.

We have one life, and we have to make it matter. But the way we chose to do it is what matters the most. Our choices make us who we are rather than our actions.

The life we live is the epitome of our intentions and morals. We can be defined in a single word or a single phrase if we ever try. We don't need to analyze someone else, we just need to see ourselves in the mirror and we might be able to see right across the image.

The day we are able to do that, might be the day we have actually made a worthy human being of ourselves and have fulfilled our destiny.

If you are able to look at yourself and go through your whole life in the blink of an eye and cherish the memories as if you were right there at that moment. Believe me, you have had a long and important life to make you think of it all over again every day.

Chapter 24:

10 Habits of Adele

There's no denying it, Adele Laurie Blue Adkins, better known as Adele is a musical legend. She is an English singer-songwriter and all-time great vocalist with excellent lyrical and passionate composing skills. Adele is one of the world's best-selling music artist, having sold over 120 million records worldwide.

With her exceptional voice and songwriting skills, the singer from a rough side of the town has captivated the hearts of millions of people. Adele got her admiration as an award-winning music legend, but moreover, there is much more from a lady who has overcome adversity to reach the top.

Here are 10 habits of Adele that will serve your learning journey.

1. It's Far From Easy

Criticism came thick and quick after Adele signed her first record deal because of her physical appearance. Many people, including Record label executives and high-profile designers publicly chastised her as "too fat" while suggesting weight loss to attract a larger fan base. Adele didn't let such criticism weigh in her talent as she unapologetically made hits after hits. Just like Adele, don't try to be anything or anyone but yourself.

2. Commitment Is Success

Despite constant pressure from the media to conform to their ludicrous notions of what women in the spotlight should look like, Adele chose her path and remained committed to being herself. This honesty is one of the attributes that Adele's fans admire. Such personality traits will breed your success.

3. It's Okay To Be Sad After a Breakup

When a relationship ends, you believe in acting tough and putting on a solid face. You're convinced on being tough to appear as you're suffering less than your ex-partners to win in some way. Adele defies expectations by telling her exes and the rest of the world about her grief without fear. She exemplifies humanity and vulnerability through her music.

4. Don't Take Life Too Seriously

It's okay to laugh at yourself or a hilarious scenario from time to time. Whether she's being teased in an interview or asked whether she wants to be a Bond Girl, Adele always respond with "Hahaha". She is quick to laugh, and her laugh is contagious.

5. Adversity Doesn't Stop Anything

Allow your pain to drive your mission. What if Adele waited till everything was back to normal before recording? All in all, people rushed to get her music, which she recorded in her misery. Every minute, every day, life happens and so should you commit to completing your projects without unconditionally.

6. Mirror Your Brand To Reflect Longevity

Say it quietly: Adele's tracks would have hit ten, twenty, or even fifty years ago. To call them timeless is a bit of a stretch. The fact may be that they're essentially personal because we believe that her music is basically from her life or personal experiences. However, Adele is always true to herself and then she sings authentically which is a formidable brand blend.

7. There Are Other Better Places Than the Spotlight

Adele doesn't constantly boost her social media presence and create "news" for constant consumption. Instead, she vanishes to do bizarre things like live and breathe and then reappears when she has something she hopes people would appreciate. It's tempting to feel the need to keep fulfilling it, but according to Adele, being true to yourself is more fulfilling.

8. Build Your Team, Not Just Yourself

When a technical issue nearly derailed her performance at Grammy Awards, Adele didn't cast an evil eye at her sound engineer. Not only did she make herself appear good by ending her performance properly, she also made her entire team look excellent. The question is, what do you do when life tosses you a curveball that you can't control?

9. Keep Going

Even when things are out of your control, it's easy to quit when everything seems to go wrong. But your perseverance will be rewarded!

10. Remember Where You Came From

Don't let your past or upbringing hold you back from achieving your goals in the future. Success is defined not by what you have as a child but by your level of commitment and work ethic over time. However, once you get there, don't forget where you come from.

Conclusion

You are characterized not by your physical appearance but by how you treat people and the words you use while communicating with everyone. Hence, just like Adele, have the confidence to pursue your aspirations. You never know where the road may take you.

Chapter 25:

8 Ways To Deal With Setbacks In Life

Life is never the same for anyone - It is an ever-changing phenomenon, making you go through all sorts of highs and lows. And as good times are an intrinsic part of your life, so are bad times. One day you might find yourself indebted by 3-digit figures while having only $40 in your savings account. Next day, you might be vacationing in Hawaii because you got a job that you like and pays $100,000 a year. There's absolutely no certainty to life (except passing away) and that's the beauty of it. You never know what is in store for you. But you have to keep living to see it for yourself. Setbacks in life cannot be avoided by anyone. Life will give you hardships, troubles, break ups, diabetes, unpaid bills, stuck toilet and so much more. It's all a part of your life.

 Here's 8 ways that you might want to take notes of, for whenever you may find yourself in a difficult position in dealing with setback in life.

1. Accept and if possible, embrace it

The difference between accepting and embracing is that when you accept something, you only believe it to be, whether you agree or disagree. But when you embrace something, you truly KNOW it to be true and accept it as a whole. There is no dilemma or disagreement after you have embraced something.

So, when you find yourself in a difficult situation in life, accept it for what it is and make yourself whole-heartedly believe that this problem in your life, at this specific time, is a part of your life. This problem is what makes you complete. This problem is meant for you and only you can go through it. And you will. Period. There can be no other way.

The sooner you embrace your problem, the sooner you can fix it. Trying to bypass it will only add upon your headaches.

2. Learn from it

Seriously, I can't emphasize how important it is to LEARN from the setbacks you face in your life. Every hardship is a learning opportunity. The more you face challenges, the more you grow. Your capabilities expand with every issue you solve—every difficulty you go through, you rediscover yourself. And when you finally deal off with it, you are reborn. You are a new person with more wisdom and experience.

When you fail at something, try to explore why you failed. Be open-minded about scrutinizing yourself. Why couldn't you overcome a certain situation? Why do you think of this scenario as a 'setback'? The moment you find the answers to these questions is the moment you will have found the solution.

3. Execute What You Have Learnt

The only next step from here is to execute that solution and make sure that the next time you face a similar situation, you'll deal with it by having both your arms tied back and blindfolded. All you have to do is remember what you did in a similar past experience and reapply your previous solution.

Thomas A. Edison, the inventor of the light bulb, failed 10,000 times before finally making it. And he said "I have not failed. I just found 10,000 ways that won't work".

The lesson here is that you have to take every setback as a lesson, that's it.

4. Without shadow, you can never appreciate light

This metaphor is applicable to all things opposite in this universe. Everything has a reciprocal; without one, the other cannot exist. Just as without shadow, we wouldn't have known what light is, similarly, without light, we could've never known about shadow. The two opposites identify and complete each other.

Too much of philosophy class, but to sum it up, your problems in life, ironically, is exactly why you can enjoy your life. For example, if you are a chess player, then defeating other chess players will give you enjoyment while getting defeated will give you distress. But, when you are a chess prodigy—you have defeated every single chess player on earth and there's no one else to defeat, then what will you do to derive pleasure? Truth is, you can now no longer enjoy chess. You have no one to defeat. No one gives you the fear of losing anymore and as a result, the taste of winning has lost its appeal to you.

So, whenever you face a problem in life, appreciate it because without it, you can't enjoy the state of not having a problem. Problems give you the pleasure of learning from them and solving them.

5. View Every Obstacle As an opportunity

This one's especially for long term hindrances to your regular life. The COVID-19 pandemic for instance, has set us back for almost two years now. As distressing it is, there is also some positive impact of it. A long-term setback opens up a plethora of new avenues for you to explore. You suddenly get a large amount of time to experiment with things that you have never tried before.

When you have to pause a regular part of your life, you can do other things in the meantime. I believe that every one of us has a specific talent and most people never know what their talent is simply because they have never tried that thing.

6. Don't Be Afraid to experiment

People pursue their whole life for a job that they don't like and most of them never ever get good at it. As a result, their true talent gets buried under their own efforts. Life just carries on with unfound potential. But when some obstacle comes up and frees you from the clutches of doing what you have been doing for a long time, then you should get around and experiment. Who knows? You, a bored high school teacher, might be a natural at tennis. You won't know it unless you are fired from that job and actually play tennis to get over it. So whenever life gives you lemons, quit trying to hold on to it. Move on and try new things instead.

7. Stop Comparing yourself to others

The thing is, we humans are emotional beings. We become emotionally vulnerable when we are going through something that isn't supposed to be. And in such times, when we see other people doing fantastic things in life, it naturally makes us succumb to more self-loathing. We think lowly of our own selves and it is perfectly normal to feel this way. Talking and comapring ourselves to people who are seemingly untouched by setbacks is a counterproductive move. You will listen to their success-stories and get depressed—lose self-esteem. Even if they try their best to advise you, it won't get through to you. You won't be able to relate to them.

8. Talk to people other people who are having their own setbacks in life

I'm not asking you to talk to just any people. I'm being very specific here: talk to people who are going through bad times as well.

If you start talking to others who are struggling in life, perhaps more so compared to you, then you'll see that everyone else is also having difficulties in life. It will seem natural to you. Moreover, having talked with others might even show you that you are actually doing better than all these other people. You can always find someone who is dealing with more trouble than you and that will enlighten you. That will encourage you. If someone else can deal with tougher setbacks in life, why can't you?

Besides, listening to other people will give you a completely new perspective that you can use for yourself if you ever find yourself in a similar situation as others whom you have talked with.

Conclusion

Setbacks are a part of life. Without them we wouldn't know what the good times are. Without them we wouldn't appreciate the success that we have gotten. Without them we wouldn't cherish the moments that got us to where we are heading to. And without them there wouldn't be any challenge to fill our souls with passion and fire. Take setbacks as a natural process in the journey. Use it to fuel your drive. Use it to move your life forward one step at a time.

Chapter 26:

How To Be A Good Public Speaker.

Public speaking is perhaps the most common and greatest fear one can endure. People would instead choose to interact with snakes or clowns than people. Just hearing about the words "public speaking" can make our palms go sweaty. But there are a hundred ways to tackle this anxiety and deliver a good speech.

Everyone undergoes physiological reactions like pounding hearts and trembling hands whenever they think about speaking publicly. Be careful to avoid associating these feelings with the sense that you might make a fool out of yourself or perform poorly. On the contrary, some nerves are good. The sweating that you get from the adrenaline rush makes you more alert, and you're then ready to give your best performance. There's no guarantee that your anxiety will completely vanish when you go to the stage facing hundreds of people, but there are ways to overcome it a little. The best way is to prepare yourself beforehand. Take your time to go over your notes. Practice a lot. Audio record or videotape yourself to see where you are lacking, get an honest friend or critique who will point out your mistakes. And once you've become comfortable with yourself, be confident and go out there!

Knowing what type of audience you're going to deal with is essential. Your audience is your main ally. Knowing and understanding them should be your priority. Engage with them by grabbing their attention. Keep the focus on them. Stay flexible and gauge their reactions. Avoid delivering a canned speech because it will only confuse or lose the attention of even the most devoted listeners.

Good communication is never flawless, and trust me; nobody even expects you to be perfect. Putting in the requisite time to prepare will help you overcome your shaky nerves and deliver a better speech. Maintain eye contact with your audience and keep the focus on yourself and your message. Keep a brief outline with you, and it can serve to jog your memory and keep you on task.

Keep thinking positively throughout your speech. It will make you feel more confident about yourself. Don't give a heads up to your fear, and it'll start a cycle of negative self-talk and self-sabotaging thoughts such as "i will start to stutter while addressing them" or "i might forget these points in nervousness." These thoughts will only lower your confidence and increase the chances of you not achieving what you're truly capable of. Affirmations and visualizations are two significant steps of improving your self-confidence. Visualize being successful in your upcoming speeches and imagine the feeling of getting done with it and leaving a positive impact on others.

Prepare yourself for any interruptions, too, and analyze how well you handle them, like sneezing in the middle of your speaking or being unprepared for a question. Do you feel surprised, hesitant, or annoyed? If you cannot handle these situations better, try to self-analyze yourself and practice managing interruptions smoothly. The next time you will get even better at dealing with stuff like that.

The more you'll get confident in public speaking, the more you will avail yourself of opportunities for success. The more you push yourself to speak in front of others, the better you will become at this. Remember, it's not a piece of cake to indulge in public speaking; the more you'll practice, the more you will excel at it. And even if it takes longer, don't doubt your ability and potential, and always be confident and believe in yourself.

Chapter 27:

6 Ways To Define What Is Important In Your Life

In this crazy world that we live in, the course of evolution spirals upward and downward, and the collective humanity has witnessed glorious times and horrific ones. The events around us change minute-to-minute. So much seems out of our control, but we find solace in knowing that one thing remains within our immediate control; taking back ownership and responsibility for ourselves. If life has gotten away from you and you feel overwhelmed, anxious or depressed, then maybe it's time to stop and refocus on what's most important to you and find a way back to what really matters to you.

The idea is to evaluate what you're actually doing with and for yourself, determine if it's even essential to you, and then make the said necessary changes that will best accommodate your needs, interests, and desires. Here are some ways to consider how and on what things you should refocus your attention to determine what is most important in your life.

1. Determine What Things You Value Most

Choose and focus on the things around which you have to structure the life that you want to create. When you consciously make these choices, you are more focused on reminding yourself what things in your life you can't and won't do without. These all represent the backbone of your life. We often forget that people and events play a massive role in shaping up to our lives. They Mold us into what we have become so far and what we are to become in the future. Their support and encouragement in our lives are undeniable. We have to see which people and what events we value the most in our lives and then should keep our focus on them more.

2. Decide What Commitments Are Essential To You

Keeping the above valuable things in mind, evaluate which commitments do you value the most in your life. Commitments are the obligations you enter into willingly and represent your promise to see any relationship/project/contract conclusion steadfastly. Renegotiate your essential commitments, if necessary, but consider completing the existing commitments that you are already obligated to and refuse to take any new ones if you aren't ready. That way, you will focus more and fulfill those commitments first that are more significant to you and your life.

3. Assess The Way You Use Your Time

Most of us have a fixed daily routine, with many fixed activities, habits, and chores. Evaluate which things are absolutely necessary and vital for shaping up your life and yourself daily. Assess the time you spend communicating, how much of your time you spend online, emailing, texting, or on your cell phone. How can you cut back the amount of time spent on these activities to do something more productive? How much time are you spending on TV, radio, reading newspapers and magazines?

Consider decreasing your consumption and receive the basic information from a reputable source only once throughout the day. Avoid repetition and redundancy.

4. Get Rid of Any clutter That's In Your Life

Look around you and see, do you need everything you have? Give away anything that you haven't used since the last two years. It could be anything, from selling items to furniture, clothing, shoes, etc. Anything that you no longer need. Someone else can happily use what you haven't all this time. And not just the worldly things; get rid of all the emotional and psychological clutter you have kept aside for so long, and it no longer serves you. We have to get rid of the old things to make room for the new things to come. This will help us reflect on our actual being of who we are and where we are.

5. Spend More Time With People That Matter To You

Evaluate how much quality time you actually spend with your family and close friends. As life evolves, more people will enter into your sphere. These people may fall into different categories of importance in your life, such as acquaintances, colleagues, friends, partners, etc. Our time is precious, so it is wise to use it on those that matter to us the most. It's necessary to sort out our interactions and to assess the meaning of each relationship to us.

6. Make Time To Be Alone

It all comes down to how much time do you make yourself at the end of the day? What was the last time you spent doing something you're passionate about or what you love doing? Give yourself all the time and permission to express your creativity and make peace with your mind. Take care of your body, spirit, and mind because these are the things that will make you feel alive. Take a walk and look around, reacquaint yourself with all the beauty around you. Make each breath count.

Conclusion

Identifying and understanding your values is a challenging but as well as an essential exercise. Your personal values are a central part of defining who you are and who you want to be. By becoming more aware of these significant factors in your life, you can use them as your best guide in any situation. It's comforting and helpful to rely on your values since most of our life's decisions are based on them.

Chapter 28:

Happy People Give Freely

"For it is in giving that we receive." - Saint Francis of Assisi.

A Chinese saying goes by, "If you want happiness for an hour, take a nap. If you want happiness for a day, go fishing. If you want happiness for a year, inherit a fortune. If you want happiness for a lifetime, help somebody." It is indeed better to give than to receive. Scientific research provides compelling anecdotal evidence that giving is a powerful pathway to personal growth and lasting happiness. When we give freely, our brain stimulates endorphins and blesses us with a feeling of euphoria. Altruism is hardwired in our brains and tends to provide us with pleasure. Helping others is a secret to living a happier and healthier, wealthier, productive, and more meaningful life.

Whether it's a charity, a piece of advice, a helping hand of any sort, or supporting someone throughout their journey, researchers Dunn, Aknin, Akin, and Norton performed a study. They showed that there is, in fact, a link between generosity and happier life. The gesture of caring about other people and doing something to improve their quality of life is the source of happiness. Once you start giving, you will feel more content and happier, and there will be no going back. You will get addicted to helping others and to the feeling that follows.

A group of psychologists from the University of California Santa Barbara conducted a study to ascertain if generosity is part of human nature. The observation showed that being a giver is more fulfilling than being a receiver and that generosity is deeply embedded in our systems. "You don't need to become a self-sacrificing martyr to feel happier. Just being a little more generous will suffice," says Prof. Tobler.

High-generosity respondents appeared not only happier but happier more often. This overarching sense of happiness in high-generosity individuals may positively affect their higher likelihood of finding life more meaningful. They were also 20% more likely to be optimistic about their future, be proud of themselves, and find enjoyment in their jobs. It's no secret that you have to give a little to get a little. The more generous you are too loved ones, acquaintances, or even strangers, the more likely those selfless deeds will be reciprocated sometime down the line. Neuroeconomics found in a recent study that merely promising to be more generous is enough to trigger a change in our brain that will eventually make us happier.

In a 2006 study, Jorge Moll and colleagues at the National Institutes of Health found that when people give, it could be anything; it activates the warm glow effect, regions of the brain associated with pleasure, social connection, and trust. Whatever you are giving to people, society, or nature, you will find yourself benefiting from a hefty dose of happiness in the process. When you express your gratitude in words or actions, you not only boost your positivity but other people's as well. The more we give, the more we stand to gain purpose, meaning, and happiness – all of the things we look for in life but are so hard to find.

Chapter 29:

Dealing with Difficult Bosses

Sometimes bosses can be A bit difficult to handle because of their expectations and behavior with the employees. But they are not impossible to deal with. You should never be discouraged by their behavior. Some people resign because of this, but in the end, the boss is not the one who is affected by this bold step, but the employee who takes this decision is affected because finding A rewarding job is never easy. There are ways to deal with difficult bosses, and by doing so, an employee can achieve big things and, at the same time, learn how to work in this environment.

The first and foremost thing to do is to evaluate the aspect because of which the boss is being difficult to work for. After that, think of the stuff that can be done to tackle that aspect. Even difficult bosses are good when you give them good results. They can be very rewarding because their expectations are always very high, so if an employee performs according to their expectations, they reward that employee generously. Some bosses get annoyed when employees skip the office or are late for work. Even in situations like illness, they are reluctant to give days off. If your boss is like this, the only thing to do is reduce your chances of illness. If A boss is target-oriented, you should be very focused on your task and should try to complete it before time to eliminate any chance of trouble. The next solution is not to be associated with groups that always cause trouble for the organization. Bosses can give A very tough time to employees who delay the targets by causing unwanted trouble.

To get the boss' attention, you should be on good terms with the managers because they are the ones who report to the leader, so by being on good terms with the managers, they will speak highly of you with the boss, and he will be happy by our attitude which can reduce the chances of behavioral problems by the boss. Increasing productivity is the key to being in the good books of A boss. In the end, it all comes to profitability which leaders care about the most. So if you are A good asset to the organization, the boss will hardly ever bother you. Also, when in direct communication with the boss, an employee should be in A very presentable manner, not only in terms of clothing but also in terms of body language and presentation skills. Words should be chosen very carefully in front of bosses. Having good communication and presenting skills is the key to getting the boss' attention in A positive way.

Some bosses are indeed difficult to work for, but by following some basic rules of thumb, employees can work without the worry of the boss being annoyed. The key is to anticipate what the leader wants from his employees, and then it comes to meeting their expectations. Employees that prove to be A valuable asset for the organization are always rewarded by the leader because such employees are the reason for the organization's success. A company can be successful only if the boss and employees are willing to work together. Even if the boss is getting on your nerves, try not to let it get to you. Recognize your importance and work hard for your own sake.

Chapter 30:

How To Design Your New Work Life

New status builds more expectations

A new job signifies many things. For the newly employed, their work status changes from unemployed to employed. It could also be a promotion to those in lower cadres when they land plum jobs. Such moments of good news are marred by happiness and confusion at the same time. Different people handle themselves differently but the common denominator is that it is a first-time experience for all of them. In a new work environment, the most common question by the new entrants is how they will manage their new work life. Are they capable of handling pressure at work or they will faint under the weight of new responsibilities? Here are a few ways of better designing a new work-life:

1. Understand your new role.

The first step as a newcomer in your new work is to know the shoes you are about to step into. What are the duties and responsibilities on your shoulders in your new capacity? You could be lucky enough to learn this in your job description or you may have to learn from those you find in the industry.

You can plan better when you are in the light of your new roles. You will not overstep your mandate when the demarcated boundaries are clear. Planning and execution of your duties will be with ease because you only operate within a laid-down framework.

Conflicts of interest can arise when the role you ought to play is unclear. Take your time to settle this with your employer. Thereafter, you can easily meet their expectations.

2. Learn the work routine.

Every workplace has its routine. What do they prioritize as they carry out their mandate? You can confirm whether or not there is an official routine to be followed in your new workplace.

Do not hesitate to seek clarification because you will be incapable of effectively discharging your duties when you are not properly briefed. Standard routines should be adhered to for you to be able to properly design your new work life.

You should also seek ways to improve the existing routines. The evolution of work routines is inevitable because of some external factors that influence them to keep on changing. You can align your new work routine in tandem with these factors such as technology and new government policies.

3. Assimilate with the existing work culture.

Work culture refers to the way an organization operates and the values it stands for. Different workplaces are founded on various values. Sometimes, the philosophy of a person could conflict with that of an organization they work for. They will have a hard time working because they do not believe in what they do.

You need to assimilate with the existing culture to properly design your new work life. Their way of doing things could be what has made them survive for a long time in the industry. Any alteration to it could wash away the gains the organization has made over time.

As a new employee, your goals should be aligned with those of the organization. You will be able to easily hit your targets and steer the company to new heights

4. Maintain professional ethics.

At the center of designing your new work-life should be professional ethics. Every job has its ethical standards that should be applied. It brings morality to the workplace. Professional ethics are tied to the worker. They should serve and work within the moral guidelines stipulated in their career.

Professional ethics should be the anchor when designing your new work life. They should guide your plans wherever you go to work. You could get a breakthrough at your new workplace when you are an ethical employee.

As you plan for better days ahead and chart a way forward in your new work life, consider professionalism above everything else. It will make you stand out from a pool of other career people.

5. Learn from experience.

Time has proven that experience is the best teacher. Those who have received their first-time employment assignment should seek the guidance of their seniors. They can guide them properly in their new work-life especially if they are in the same profession.

Those who have moved from one organization to another can use the experience in their previous workstation to settle in their new work life. The best form of learning is from the mistakes of other people instead of yours.

In conclusion, designing your new work-life involves consideration of many factors. These are the five primary ones you should consider implementing.

Chapter 31:

10 Habits of Angela Merkel

Angela Dorothea Merkel is the first female in the history of Germany to become a chancellor. She is known as a de facto leader of the European Union and the most powerful woman for a decade. She has been serving as Chancellor of Germany for 16 years and has no plans to seek another term this year.

Angela Merkel is one of only two EU leaders to have survived the economic crisis, a migrant crisis, the Euro debt crisis, as well as the Covid-19 pandemic; she has triumphed. Her leadership is realistic and organized; a person who has shunned risky decisions and sought a middle ground. Her principles, kindness, resilience- helped her establish moral leadership in a world of disputed patriarchy. So what are the secrets to her success?

Here are 10 Habits of Angela Merkel.

1. Be Practical and Methodical

You don't need a scientific mentality to know the rigors of a planned economy. It's mainly about your character; what matters more for Merkel is the structure and avoiding chaos. She claims her job is "advancing and solving issues even if it's a few centimetres away."

2. Know What Your Country Needs

When the opportunity to go to battle arises, could you not take it? Especially when your people adamantly oppose. Just play it safe on Iraq; commit only your bare minimum to Afghanistan, and reject participation in Libya and Syria. That Merkel!

3. Gender Is Not a Limit

Governance is a way of life, not a gender trait, and anytime you doubt a female's ability to govern, take a cue from Merkel. Her leadership story in one of the most advanced nations is a true example of women's empowerment. She has demonstrated to the world that your potential and character, rather than gender, defines a leader.

4. Resilience

Leaders would seem phony without resilience. When you strive to bring change as a leader, you'll have people trying to oust you from the spotlight. However, your strength and perseverance will shine you through. Merkel joined politics in 1989 and has been an active opposition leader for many years. Her resilient personality paid off in 2005, hence proving wrong those who questioned her potential.

5. Visionary

Being a great orator or a socialist isn't enough for leadership. You need a vision! Why did Merkel win four consecutive terms? She is a true prowess and charm of a visionary person. Her dream was to attain and sustain a powerful position for Germany's economy and environmental role. Today, Germany comes fourth among the advanced global economies.

6. Her Altruistic Traits

When you are arrogant and self-centered as a leader, you will not last more than two terms. Angela Merkel's selfless devotion to serving Germany for developmental objectives gave her a competitive edge over her adversaries. She is regarded as a fine endorser of democratic leadership.

7. A Critical Thinker

Few leaders in Europe are as deft as Merkel. She knows how to handle the menacing threat of Vladimir Putin's Russia while also ensuring the Greeks remain in the European Union. She is a critical thinker who has proved that when you put on a strategic plan, relying on informed information, you'll overcome problems without going to war.

8. Know When to Quit

After becoming the longest-serving head of government, Merkel early this year decided not to vie for another term. Staying in power and never leaving the stage can spoil the work you have already done.

9. Have a Strategy – But Never Divulge It

The ideal move to achieving anything is by keeping your plans or ideologies a secret. That is, seek and achieve your goals in secret. There was purportedly Merkel's strategy to save Euro on a single piece of paper. But did she ever reveal her plan? She's a heck. She got criticized as a bad public speaker, but it worked for her.

10. Show Gratitude

While fighting and preventing the spread of Corona Virus, and after her solidarity statement and flattening curve explanation, Merkel gave a heartfelt thank you to medical practitioners, acknowledging their sacrifice and hard work on behalf of everyone else. Always portray unquestionable gratitude to those who help make your leadership manageable.

Conclusion

Every great leader is an exceptional teacher, and Angela Merkel is no exception. From her resiliency to her humanitarian attitude, she exemplifies many leadership qualities that you can learn from. She is living proof that you can achieve anything in life when you have aspirations and put on your courage to pursue them.

Chapter 32:

8 Ways To Love Yourself First

"Your task is not to seek for love, but merely to seek and find all the barriers within yourself that you have built against it." - Rumi.

Most of us are so busy waiting for someone to come into our lives and love us that we have forgotten about the one person we need to love the most – ourselves. Most psychologists agree that being loved and being able to love is crucial to our happiness. As quoted by Sigmund Freud, "love and work … work and love. That's all there is." It is the mere relationship of us with ourselves that sets the foundation for all other relationships and reveals if we will have a healthy relationship or a toxic one.

Here are some tips on loving yourself first before searching for any kind of love in your life.

1. Know That Self-Love Is Beautiful

Don't ever consider self-love as being narcissistic or selfish, and these are two completely different things. Self-love is rather having positive regard for our wellbeing and happiness. When we adopt self-love, we see higher levels of self-esteem within ourselves, are less critical and harsh with ourselves while making mistakes, and can celebrate our positive qualities and accept all our negative ones.

2. Always be kind to yourself:

We are humans, and humans are tended to get subjected to hurts, shortcomings, and emotional pain. Even if our family, friends, or even our partners may berate us about our inadequacies, we must learn to accept ourselves with all our imperfections and flaws. We look for acceptance from others and be harsh on ourselves if they tend to be cruel or heartless with us. We should always focus on our many positive qualities, strengths, and abilities, and admirable traits; rather than harsh judgments, comparisons, and self-hatred get to us. Always be gentle with yourself.

3. Be the love you feel within yourself:

You may experience both self-love and self-hatred over time. But it would be best if you always tried to focus on self-love more. Try loving yourself and having positive affirmations. Do a love-kindness meditation or spiritual practices to nourish your soul, and it will help you feel love and compassion toward yourself. Try to be in that place of love throughout your day and infuse this love with whatever interaction you have with others.

4. Give yourself a break:

We don't constantly live in a good phase. No one is perfect, including ourselves. It's okay to not be at the top of your game every day, or be happy all the time, or love yourself always, or live without pain. Excuse your bad days and embrace all your imperfections and mistakes. Accept your negative emotions but don't let them overwhelm you. Don't set high standards for yourself, both emotionally and mentally. Don't judge yourself for whatever you feel, and always embrace your emotions wholeheartedly.

5. Embrace yourself:

Are you content to sit all alone because the feelings of anxiety, fear, guilt, or judgment will overwhelm you? Then you have to practice being comfortable in your skin. Go within and seek solace in yourself, practice moments of alone time and observe how you treat yourself. Allow yourself to be mindful of your beliefs, feelings, and thoughts, and embrace solitude. The process of loving yourself starts with understanding your true nature.

6. Be grateful:

Rhonda Bryne, the author of The Magic, advises, "When you are grateful for the things you have, no matter how small they may be, you will see those things instantly increase." Look around you and see all the things that you are blessed to have. Practice gratitude daily and be thankful for all the things, no matter how good or bad they are. You will immediately start loving yourself once you realize how much you have to be grateful for.

7. Be helpful to those around you:

You open the door for divine love the moment you decide to be kind and compassionate toward others. "I slept and dreamt that life was a joy. I awoke and saw that life was service. I acted, and behold, and service was a joy." - Rabindranath Tagore. The love and positive vibes that you wish upon others and send out to others will always find a way back to you. Your soul tends to rejoice when you are kind, considerate, and compassionate. You have achieved the highest form of self-love when you decide to serve others. By helping others, you will realize that you don't need someone else to feel complete; you are complete. It will help you feel more love and fulfillment in your life.

8. Do things you enjoy doing:

If you find yourself stuck in a monotonous loop, try to get some time out for yourself and do the things that you love. There must be a lot of hobbies and passions that you might have put a brake on. Dust them off and start doing them again. Whether it's playing any sport, learning a new skill, reading a new book, writing in on your journal, or simply cooking or baking for yourself, start doing it again. We shouldn't compromise on the things that make us feel alive. Doing the things we enjoy always makes us feel better about ourselves and boost our confidence.

Conclusion:

Loving yourself is nothing short of a challenge. It is crucial for your emotional health and ability to reach your best potential. But the good news is, we all have it within us to believe in ourselves and live the best life we possibly can. Find what you are passionate about, appreciate yourself, and be grateful for what's in your life. Accept yourself as it is.

Chapter 33:

Five Steps to Clarify Your Goals

Today, we're going to talk about how and why you should start clarifying your goals.

But first, let me ask you, why do you think setting clear goals is important?

Well, imagine yourself running at a really fast speed, but you don't know where you're going. You just keep running and running towards any direction without a destination in mind. What do you think will happen next? You'll be exhausted. But will you feel fulfilled? Not really. Why? Because despite running at breakneck speed and being busy, you have failed to identify an end point. Without it, you won't know how far or near you are to where you are supposed to be. The same analogy applies to how we live our lives. No matter how productive you are or how fast your pacing is, at the end the race, if you don't have clear goals, you will simply end up wondering what the whole point of running was in the first place. You might end up in a place that you didn't intend to be. Neglecting the things that are most important on you, while focusing on all the wrong things- and that is not the best way to live your life.

So, how can we change that? How can we clarify our goals so that we are sure that we are running the race we intended to all along?

1. Imagine The Ideal Version of Yourself

Try to picture the kind of person you want to be. The things you want to have. The people you want around you. The kind of life that your ideal self is living. How does your ideal-self make small and big decisions? How does he or she perceive the world? Don't limit your imagination to what you think is pleasant and acceptable in society.

Fully integrate that ideal image of yourself into your subconscious mind and see yourself filling those shoes. That is the only way that you'll be able to see it as a real person.

Remember that the best version of yourself doesn't need to be perfect. But this is your future life so dream as big as you want, and genuinely believe that you'll be able to become that person someday in the near future.

2. Identify The Gap Between Your Ideal and Present Self

Take a hard look at your current situation now and ask yourself honesty: "How far am I away now from the person I know I need to become one day? What am I lacking at present that I am not doing or acting upon? Are there any areas that I can identify that I need to work on? Are there any new habits that I need to adopt to become that person?

Be unbiased in your self-assessment as that is the only way to give yourself a clear view of knowing exactly what you need to start working on today. Be brutally honest with your self-evaluation.

It is okay to be starting from scratch if that is where are at this point. Don't be afraid of the challenge, instead embrace and prepare yourself for the journey of a lifetime. It is way worse not knowing when and where to begin than starting from nothing at all.

3. Start Making Your Action Plan

Once you have successfully identified the gap between your present self and your ideal self, start to list down all the actions you need to take and the things that need to be done. Breakdown your action plan into milestones. Make it specific, measurable and realistic. If your action plans don't work the way you think they will, don't be afraid to make new plans. Remember that your failed plans are just part of the whole journey so enjoy every moment of it. Don't be hard on yourself while you're in the process. You're a human and not a machine. Don't forget to rest and recharge from time to time. You will be more inspired and will have more energy to go through your action plan if you are taking care of yourself at   the   same   time.

4.   Set A Timeline

Now that you have identified your overarching goal and objectives, set a period of time when you think it is reasonable for a certain milestone to be completed. You don't need to be so rigid with this timeline. Instead use it as sort of a guiding light. This guide is to serve as a reminder to provide a sense of urgency to work on your goals consistently. Don't beat yourself up unnecessarily if you do not meet your milestones as you have set up. Things change and problems do come up in our lives. As long as you keep going, you're perfectly fine. Remember that it is not about how slow or how fast you get to your destination, it is about how you persevere to continue your journey.

5. Aim For Progress, Not Perfection

You are living in an imperfect world with an imperfect system. Things will never be perfect but it doesn't mean that it will be less beautiful. While you're in the process of making new goals and working on them as you go along, always make room for mistakes and adjustments. You can plan as much as you want but life has its own way of doing things. When unforeseen events take place, don't be afraid to make changes and adjustments, or start over if you must. Even though things will not always go the way you want them to, you can still be in control of choosing how you'll move forward.

As humans, we never want to be stuck. We always want to be somewhere better. But sometimes, we get lost along the way. If we have a clear picture of where we want to be, no matter how many detours we encounter, we'll always find our way to get to our destination. And you know what, sometimes those detours are what we exactly need to keep going through our journey.

Chapter 34:

How Getting Out of Your Comfort Zone Could Be The Best Thing Ever

A comfort zone is best described as the place where you feel comfortable and your abilities are not being tested, or a place where you don't have to try anything new or different. We have all heard the advice of getting out of our comfort zone. Its sure sounds like an easy phrase, but any advice is easier to give than to take. While it is true that the ability to take risks by stepping outside your comfort zone is the primary way by which we grow, it's also true that we are often afraid to take that first step. Embracing new experiences can bloom your life and could even change the direction of your career. Comfort zones are not really about comfort; and they are about fear. So, break the chains and step out; you will enjoy the process of taking risks and growing. Here are some ways to get out of your comfort zone to experience a better life.

1. Become Aware Of What's Outside The Comfort Zone

You believe so many things are worth doing, but the thought of disappointment and failure always holds you back. Identify the things that you are afraid of doing and assess the discomforts associated with them. Start working on them slowly and gradually. You will see how much progress you will make and how much you will grow following that. Once your discomforts no longer scare you, you will see how confident you will become in trying new things.

2. Have A Clear Sight About What You Have To Overcome

There would be many situations that get you anxious and uncomfortable. Please make a list of all of them and go deeper. The primary emotion associated with all of our negative thoughts that we try to overcome is fear. Are you afraid of public speaking because you are insecure about your voice? Do you get nervous around people and avoid talking to them for fear of being ignored? Be specific in your areas of discomfort, and then work on your insecurities to get more confident.

3. Get Comfortable With Discomfort

Expand your comfort zone to get out of it. Make it your goal to stop running away from the discomforts. If you can't make eye contact while talking, try locking it a bit more rather than immediately looking out. If you stay long enough and practice it, it will start to become less uncomfortable.

4. See Failure As A Teacher

Many of us are so scared of failures that we would prioritize doing absolutely nothing other than taking a shot at our dreams and goals. We have to treat our failures as a teacher. We learn more from failures than we do from successes. Take that experience that has caused you to fail and evaluate how you can take that lesson your next time so that the chance of success increases. Many of the world's famous people, and even billionaires and millionaires, failed the thousandth time before succeeding.

5. Take Baby Steps

Don't try to achieve everything at once. If you jump outside your comfort zone, the chances are that you will become overwhelmed and jump right back in. Always start by taking small steps, overcome the fear of little things first. It's the small steps along the journey that ensures our extraordinary destination. If you are afraid of public speaking, start by speaking to a smaller group of people or even your family and friends. This will help you built self-confidence, and you will be ready to talk on public platforms in no time.

6. Hang out with risk-takers:

If you want to become better at something, start hanging out with people who already took the risk, who already are doing the things you planned to do. Start emulating them. No one can give you the best insight into the situations than those who already have experienced it. Almost inevitably, their influence will start affecting your behavior, and you too will get a clear mind about things.

7. Be Honest With Yourself

Stop making excuses for the things that you are too afraid to do. You might be tricking your brain into thinking that maybe you don't have enough time to do your tasks. But in reality, you are scared of giving it a chance and risking failure. Don't make excuses but instead, be honest. You will be in a better place to confront what is truly bothering you, and this will increase your chance of moving forward.

8. Identify New Opportunities

Staying in your comfort zone is like sitting in a closed room or wearing blinders. You will convince yourself that you already dislike the things you didn't even try yet and only care about the already part of your life. But you have to put your walls down, not thickens them, and take risks. You will be amazed at how many opportunities you will be exposed to when you finally let yourself out.

Conclusion

It will seem scary at first to get out of your comfort zone, but it will be the best experience of your life. Don't jump right out of it; slowly push yourself past your comfort zone. You will eventually feel more and more comfortable about the new stuff you were too afraid to try.

www.ingramcontent.com/pod-product-compliance
Lightning Source LLC
Chambersburg PA
CBHW050737030426
42336CB00012B/1617